Guide to Cannabis

*Learn about the science behind cannabis and the
many different uses for the plant.*

As the use for cannabis as medicine becomes more and
more mainstream, it is important to know the facts behind
the plant.

In this revolutionary Itty Bitty® Book, Dr. Hyla Cass and
Mikayla Kemp explore the science, uses and
administration methods for using cannabis.

In this book, you will learn all of the basics of the
cannabis plant to help you make a more informed
decision about using cannabis for your health.

For example:

- Learn about the different parts of the plant and
  the different chemicals found within the plant.
- Understand how different cannabinoids and
  terpenes interact with your body.
- Grasp the different administration methods, and
  why certain methods are better for specific
  ailments.

Pick up a copy of this informative book today and
become educated on the health benefits of this plant that
everyone is talking about.

Your Amazing Itty Bitty® Guide to Cannabis

15 Key Steps to Understanding the Many Benefits of the Cannabis Plant

Hyla Cass M.D. &
Mikayla Kemp

Published by Itty Bitty® Publishing
A subsidiary of S & P Productions, Inc.

Copyright © 2018 **Hyla Cass M.D. & Mikayla Kemp**

Printed in the United States of America

Itty Bitty® Publishing
311 Main Street, Suite D
El Segundo, CA 90245
(310) 640-8885

ISBN: 978-0-9992211-6-7

Table of Contents

Introduction
Step 1.   Cannabis, What Is That?
Step 2.   Common Misconceptions
Step 3.   Sativa And Indica
Step 4.   THC
Step 5.   CBD
Step 6.   Terpenes
Step 7.   The Entourage Effect
Step 8.   The Endocannabinoid System
Step 9.   Smoking
Step 10.   Vaping
Step 11.   Edibles
Step 12.   Sublingual
Step 13.   Topical
Step 14.   Transdermal
Step 15.   Testing

Stop by our Itty Bitty® website to find interesting information regarding cannabis education.

Visit Hyla Cass M.D. & Mikayla Kemp at

Cassmd.com (Dr. Cass)
CannabisForWellness.org (Mikayla)

Introduction

Welcome to your guide to cannabis! This book aims to go over a broad explanation of the cannabis plant, its many benefits, as well as different administration methods. Both authors feel strongly that if used correctly and responsibly, cannabis can be used to help treat many different ailments.

Quick reference guide:

Cannabis: Genus name for the plant commonly known as marijuana.

Trichomes: Glands found on the flowers that release both cannabinoids and terpenes.

Cannabinoids: Chemicals found specifically in cannabis and responsible for many of the effects of cannabis.

Terpenes: Chemicals found within many plants that are responsible for the smell of the plant.

*Note: The citations for the studies mentioned in this book can be found by going to CannabisForWellness.org/guide-to-cannabis

Step 1
Cannabis, What Is That?

Cannabis, pot, weed, marijuana, etc., are all the same thing, but since it is important to view this as a plant with medicinal value rather than a type of illicit drug, it will be referred to as cannabis in this book.

1. Unfortunately, there have been years of stigma and negative propaganda that have shaped a belief around cannabis that is simply untrue.
2. Cannabis has been proven time and time again to produce many different therapeutic and medicinal effects, including, but not limited to:
   a. pain management,
   b. nausea control,
   c. anti-inflammatory properties,
   d. neuroprotective properties,
   e. and many more.

Cannabis, What Is That?

Therapeutic and medicinal properties are not the only benefit of cannabis. Cannabis can be grown organically and all parts of the plant can be used.

- A cannabis plant typically takes up to 6 months to fully mature to a time of harvest.
- The dried flower portions of the plant are what are most commonly used for medicinal purposes because they contain the trichomes, the shiny crystalline factories that produce the hundreds of known <u>cannabinoids</u>, terpenes, and flavonoids.
- The stalk can be used to create textiles for clothing, as well as industrial textiles for rope and carpets. It can also be used to make paper products, and much more.
- Leaves can be used for anything from juicing to animal bedding.
- Ever see hemp seeds in the grocery store? These seeds can be used as dietary fiber, as well as for their oil.
- The roots can be used in compost.

Step 2
Common Misconceptions

There are many misconceptions that surround cannabis use, mostly due to the negative stigma about the plant. The common misconceptions are listed below:

1. Only stoners use cannabis.
2. Cannabis makes you lazy.
3. Smoking is the only way to use cannabis.
4. You need to get high to benefit from cannabis.

All the above statements are false, but are commonly believed by individuals who are not fully educated on cannabis and cannabis use.

Common Misconceptions

Only Stoners Use Cannabis.
- *All* types of people use cannabis. This ranges from professionals to athletes to elderly individuals. People use cannabis for many different reasons.

Cannabis Makes You Lazy.
- While there are cases of misuse and individuals becoming a "lazy stoner," this does not apply across the board. The result of cannabis use depends on the full chemical profile of the strain and the individual's desired outcome.

Smoking Is the Only Way to Use Cannabis.
- There are many different methods of administration, so that if someone wanted to use cannabis, but did not want to smoke, they could receive the benefits a different way.

You Need To Get High To Benefit From Cannabis.
- The benefits of cannabis are not related to the psychoactive ingredient THC or tetrahydrocannabinol. There are many different chemicals found in cannabis that are quite effective and don't get you high.

Step 3
Sativa and Indica

Shopping for cannabis can be overwhelming if you do not fully understand what you are looking for. Commonly, different strains are labeled as Sativa or Indica. A common belief is that a Sativa plant is more uplifting and an Indica plant is more sedating. While this may be partially true, there are many studies that suggest that the effect of the plant is based more on the full chemical profile. Sativa and Indica refer more to the *type* of cannabis plant and the plant's physical appearance.

1. Sativa plants are tall with thin leaves.
2. Indica plants are short and bushy with thicker leaves.
3. A hybrid plant is a plant that is a crossbreed between two different types of plants.

Sativa and Indica

Have you ever gone into a dispensary and purchased a Sativa, but the effect ended up feeling more like what you would have imagined an Indica to feel like? You are not alone.

- There are many different types of cannabinoids found in the cannabis plant.
- Different percentages of these cannabinoids have a large effect on how the strain will affect you.
- Cannabis also contains chemicals called terpenes which have their own therapeutic effects.
- Different types and percentages of terpenes can be responsible for how the strain of cannabis affects you.

Many factors can affect the cannabinoid and terpene levels in the different strains of cannabis, including climate, weather, time of harvest, type of fertilizer and soil type. So, the same strain grown at different times of the year in different locations can have *slightly* different chemical profiles resulting in *slightly* different effects.

What to take away from this? KNOW the chemical profile of the strain.

Step 4
THC

THC or Tetrahydrocannabinol is the most commonly known cannabinoid and usually the most prevalent one in cannabis. THC is the cannabinoid that is responsible for the psychoactive effects or the "high."

1. THC is known for getting someone high.
2. THC is not only useful for the "high," but is also responsible for many different therapeutic effects which include:
   a. Reduction of nausea and vomiting
   b. Reduction of pain
   c. Muscle relaxation
   d. Stimulation of appetite

THC

Reduction of Nausea and Vomiting.
- A 2015 study suggested that the use of THC dramatically decreased vomiting and stomach retching in small mammals.

Reduction of Pain.
- A 2015 journal review examined randomized, controlled trials where cannabinoids, including THC, were used as treatment for chronic pain. The authors found cannabis to be a safe and effective option for managing pain.

Muscle Relaxation.
- A 2012 study outlined the outcome of a trial for cannabis to help treat muscle spasms due to Multiple Sclerosis (MS). The trial demonstrated that participants who got the cannabis attained a rate of relief from muscle stiffness that was almost twice that of those receiving the placebo.

Stimulation of Appetite.
- This might not sound therapeutic to everyone, but for an individual struggling with weight loss due to cancer, AIDS or anorexia, this could mean everything.

Step 5
CBD

CBD or Cannabidiol is another cannabinoid found in the cannabis plant. Unlike THC, this cannabinoid produces little to no psychoactive effect. CBD is the go-to cannabinoid for someone looking for therapeutic effects without the traditional "high."

1. CBD can be administered in all of the same ways that THC can. Products can contain only CBD or a ratio of CBD: THC. The ideal ratio depends on the individual's body chemistry, as well as the desired effect.
2. CBD contains many different medicinal and therapeutic properties. The most common known properties are below:
    a. Anti-anxiety
    b. Anti-epileptic
    c. Neuro-protective
    d. Anti-inflammatory
    e. Analgesic
    f. Anti-tumor

CBD

Anti-anxiety
- CBD oil was found to be a safe treatment for reducing anxiety and helping to improve sleep in young girls.

Anti-epileptic
- CBD has shown significant anticonvulsant effects in small animals and the data that we do have has shown tremendous promise in helping both children and adults.

Neuroprotective
- CBD could provide neuroprotection due to its oxidative properties, potentially helping in neurodegenerative disorders.

Anti-inflammatory
- It has been shown that CBD reduced cytokine levels, in turn, reducing inflammation.

Analgesic
- CBD by itself is used mostly for inflammatory pain, but has promising effects on chronic and neuropathic pain when utilized with THC.

Anti-tumor
- CBD has been shown to stop or slow down the growth and spread of cancer cells, likely because of CBD's ability to increase oxidative stress on cancer cells.

Step 6
Terpenes

A large variety of essential oils are used for their therapeutic effects. These plant oils are comprised largely of terpenes, chemicals that give them their unique aromas. Cannabis contains many different healing terpenes, with various strains having different types and concentrations of terpenes— and thence their own distinctive smells.

1. Terpenes contain their own properties, included, but not limited to: anti-inflammatory, anti-anxiety, pain management, sleep aid and antidepressant.
2. Common terpenes found in cannabis are:
   a. Alpha-pinene
   b. Linalool
   c. Beta-caryophyllene
   d. Myrcene
   e. Limonene

\

Terpenes

Alpha-pinene
- Present in pine needles, conifers and sage with a pine-like aroma. The terpene is understood to be anti-inflammatory, a bronchodilator and can help combat memory loss.

Linalool
- Commonly found in lavender, laurel, birch and rosewood, producing a floral scent. This terpene is understood to contain calming and sedating properties.

Beta-caryophyllene
- Present in cloves, basil, oregano, and pepper, with a pepper and spice type of aroma. This terpene is known to have antioxidant and anti-inflammatory properties, as well as aiding in sleep.

Myrcene
- Commonly found in mango, thyme and bay leaves, with a musty, herbal aroma. This terpene is known to contain anti-bacterial, anti-fungal and anti-inflammatory properties. Myrcene is known to be partially responsible for the sedative effects in certain strains.

Limonene
- Commonly found in citrus and peppermint with a citrusy aroma. This terpene is known to contain anti-depressant and anti-anxiety properties.

Step 7
The Entourage Effect

The Entourage Effect is described as cannabinoids and terpenes working together to produce a stronger therapeutic effect than if they were working alone.

1. Many studies have shown that full plant extract or extracts containing multiple cannabinoids have been more beneficial than just THC alone.
2. Different cannabinoids work together to produce different types of effects.
3. Terpenes and cannabinoids also work together to produce therapeutic effects.

The Entourage Effect

Full Plant Extract.
- Full plant extract is an extract that contains all the cannabinoids and terpenes extracted from a plant rather than just an isolated cannabinoid.

Cannabinoids Working with Other Cannabinoids.
- CBD is commonly known to decrease the psychoactive effects of THC.
- CBD can also prolong the effects of THC by slowing down the degradation of THC in the liver.

Cannabinoids Working with Terpenes.
- A 2013 study suggested that cannabinoids used in combination with beta-caryophyllene are shown to be a promising candidate for the treatment of chronic pain.
- It has been suggested that pinene and THC together have potential effects in helping Alzheimer's patients due both to the neuroprotective properties of THC and Pinene's ability to help combat memory loss.

Step 8
The Endocannabinoid System

The Endocannabinoid System (ECS) is a system within our bodies that both directly and indirectly interacts with endocannabinoids and phytocannabinoids.

The ECS helps regulate the following:
1. Appetite
2. Sleep
3. Energy
4. Balance
5. Mood
6. Stress
7. Muscle spasticity
8. Neurogenesis
9. Pain

The ECS also potentially helps regulate the following:
1. The immune system
2. Tumor surveillance
3. Fertility
4. Bone physiology

The ECS has different components, including:
1. Endocannabinoids
2. Receptors
3. Regulatory Enzymes

The Endocannabinoid System

Endocannabinoids
- These are cannabinoids that are made in the body and interact with the same receptors as phytocannabinoids, cannabinoids found in cannabis.

Receptors
- Think of receptors as the lock and cannabinoids as the key. Cannabinoids, both endo- and phyto- interact with the receptors creating different outcomes.
- CB_1 receptors are one type of receptor in the ECS. These receptors are the main psychoactive receptor.
- CB_2 receptors are the other known receptor in the ECS. CB_2 is primarily responsible for immunomodulatory and anti-inflammatory properties.

Regulatory Enzymes
- Enzymes are proteins in our body that regulate chemical reactions.
- The enzymes involved in the ECS either create endocannabinoids or break them down.

Step 9
Smoking

There are many different ways that cannabis can be administered. Smoking is one of the most common and well-known. It is always good to learn the various types of administration methods available, as some are better than others for certain ailments or effects.

1. Smoking cannabis produces combustion.
2. There are different methods of smoking cannabis.
3. There are both benefits and concerns in smoking cannabis.

Smoking Methods
1. Joint – Cannabis flower that is rolled using rolling papers.
2. Bubbler – A small water pipe that allows for smaller hits while still passing the smoke through water.
3. Pipe – Typically made of glass and acts as a vessel for the smoke to move from the lit flower into the mouth of the user.
4. Bong – A larger waterpipe that passes the smoke through water which helps it cool down and filters out some smoke toxins.

Smoking

Combustion is the process of burning something. The combustion occurs when you light the cannabis flower on fire.

Benefits
- There is a very quick onset of effects, usually occurring around 90 seconds.
- If the smoke is passed through the water, some smoke toxins are filtered, but not all.

Concerns
- Inhaling any type of smoke causes harmful irritants and carcinogens to enter the lungs.
- The tar related to the smoke is not removed by passing through a water pipe.

Step 10
Vaping

Vaping is similar to smoking in the sense that you are inhaling the cannabis, but it does not create any combustion. Vaping uses warm air or heat, rather than a flame.

1. Vaping creates similar effects to smoking cannabis.
2. Vaping is sometimes thought of as the healthier option, but there are some concerns.
3. Temperature-controlled vaporizers are very important.

Vaping

When vaping, the temperatures should be between 180° and 200° Celsius to ensure that vaporization is occurring instead of combustion.

Benefits
- Vaping creates a quick onset of effects, typically within 90 seconds.
- Vaping *should* be a smokeless delivery, but only if done properly.

Concerns
- If the temperature is too high, there is a chance that combustion is occurring and you are inhaling smoke instead of vapor.
- Some products say they are vaporizers, but there is no way to determine the temperature they are using.
- There are also some products on the market that contain temperature control systems that you are able to set to guarantee you are receiving vapor.

Step 11
Edibles

Edibles refer to anything containing cannabis products that you ingest and pass through your digestive system.

1. Edibles have a much longer onset time than smoking or vaping.
2. Around 50% of the THC that you ingest turns into 11-hydroxy-THC by the liver cells before it enters the bloodstream.
3. There are both benefits and concerns when it comes to using edibles.

Edibles

Edibles are great for longer lasting effects, but are not the best administration method for the treatment of nausea and vomiting. The onset of edibles occurs approximately 90 minutes after ingestion, depending on individual body chemistry.

Benefits
- There is no combustion or irritation to the lungs.
- Edibles produce a longer lasting effect, from around 4-12 hours, depending on the dose.

Concerns
- The metabolite, 11-hydroxy-THC, is about 4-times more psychoactive than THC. This creates a higher possibility of over-consumption than any of the other administration methods.
- The effects depend on the individuals body chemistry, so the effects vary from person to person.
- Using edibles can be difficult for patients who are anorexic, nauseous or vomiting.
- Make sure you read the ingredients, since many edibles contain high amounts of sugar or other unhealthy ingredients. There are brands on the market, however, that do create healthy edibles.

Step 12
Sublingual or Oromucosal

Sublingual refers to a cannabis tincture or oil being absorbed through the mucous membrane under your tongue. There are also oromucosal sprays that are absorbed through the mucous membrane of your cheeks.

1. The onset is faster than edibles but slower than smoking or vaping.
2. The levels of the cannabinoids in the bloodstream are typically lower than after inhalation from smoking or vaping.
3. There are both benefits and concerns to sublingual or oromucosal administration.

Sublingual or Oromucosal

Benefits

- Passing through the mucous membrane allows cannabinoids to go directly into the bloodstream and not pass through your gastrointestinal tract.
- The onset of effects usually occurs in around 30 minutes, but can vary depending on the individual's body chemistry.
- This method of administration is much more desirable than edibles for treating nausea and vomiting, as it is absorbed instead of swallowed.

Concerns

- Most of the tincture or spray should be absorbed through the mucous membrane, but sometimes part of the medication is swallowed.
- If it is swallowed, it will pass through gastrointestinal tract and have a slightly different effect.
- How much was swallowed and how much was absorbed can affect both the strength of the medication and the time of its onset.

Step 13
Topical

Topicals are cannabis products that are commonly found in the form of creams, balms and salves. Topicals work best for localized treatment for pain and inflammation.

1. Topicals are typically non-psychoactive.
2. The cannabinoids bind to the CB_2 receptors closer to the surface of the skin.
3. The cannabinoids in topicals, unlike transdermals, typically do not enter the bloodstream in high concentrations.

Topical

Benefits
- Topicals are a great administration method for an individual who does not want to experience any psychoactive effects.
- The cannabinoids and terpenes contained in the topical are typically only able to reach the CB_2 receptors, which are predominantly responsible for immunomodulatory and anti-inflammatory effects.
- Even if the topical contains THC, the cannabinoid should not enter the bloodstream and instead will produce therapeutic effects with the CB_2 receptors rather than the CB_1 receptors.

Concerns
- The concerns with topicals are minimal, as experiencing too much of a "high" from them is virtually impossible.
- Topicals are not the best administration method for someone experiencing nausea and vomiting or who requires cannabinoids binding to the CB_1 receptors in the central nervous system.

Step 14
Transdermal

Transdermal administration and topical administration are commonly used interchangeably, which is incorrect. Unlike topical administration, transdermal allows for the cannabinoids and terpenes to enter into the bloodstream, which allows for the cannabinoids and terpenes to reach the CB_1 receptors in the central nervous system. Transdermal products come in the form of patches.

1. Transdermal patches allow cannabinoids and terpenes to enter the bloodstream.
2. Patches often come in different ratios of cannabinoids so an individual can choose which dose is correct for them.

Transdermal

Benefits

- The transdermal patches often contain a carrier which helps bring the cannabinoids through the skin and into the bloodstream.
- The transdermal patches can produce psychoactive effects, so many companies create patches that come with different ratios. These ratios allow the individual to choose which cannabinoids and in what concentration they want to receive them.
- Not *all* transdermal patches produce a psychoactive effect.

Concerns

- People often mix up topical and transdermal, so there is a concern that an individual who does not want to experience psychoactive effects uses a transdermal patch instead of a topical and experiences an effect they were not anticipating.

Step 15
Testing

Viewing the lab analysis for the cannabis products that you purchase is incredibly important. Many companies provide these test results right on the packaging or upon request. You want to view testing results for two main reasons: what are the cannabinoids and terpenes present in the products and is there anything in the product that should not be there?

1. Look for the types of cannabinoids and terpenes present, as well as how prevalent they are in the product.
2. Look out for pesticides, mold or residual solvents.

Testing

Cannabinoids and Terpenes

- The full effects of the cannabis product are determined by the chemical profile of the specific plant that was used to create it.
- Knowing which cannabinoids and terpenes are in the product, as well as their concentration, can give you a better idea of the effect to help guide your purchasing.

Pesticides, Mold, and Residual Solvents

- There are not always regulations on how to grow cannabis plants, so understanding if your flower has been grown using pesticides or not is incredibly important.
- There can sometimes be mold on the plant while it grows. Many companies will get rid of the batch that carries mold, but sometimes it is hard to see. A negative result for mold is important for health.
- Residual solvents are solvents that are left in the concentrate after the extraction process. Examples are butane, hexane, and propane, which are all solvents that you do not want in your extract. There are solvent-free extraction processes as well.

You've finished. Before you go...

<u>Tweet/share that you finished this book.</u>

Please star rate this book.

Reviews are solid gold to writers. Please take a few minutes to give us some itty bitty feedback.

ABOUT THE AUTHORS

Mikayla Kemp has a B.S. in Biology from Loyola Marymount University where she performed genetic and evolutionary research and was inducted into Sigma Xi, the Scientific Research Society. Education being her passion, she quickly became the Science Department Head at a middle and high school in Los Angeles. She later joined a prominent cannabis company where she ran the training department for a year. Since then, her own company, Cannabis for Wellness, has consulted with various clients, educating them on general cannabis use and on specific products to help with their ailments. http://cannabisforwellness.org

Hyla Cass, MD is a psychiatrist and frequently quoted expert in the area of natural approaches to mental and physical health. She combines the best of leading-edge natural medicine with modern science in her clinical practice, writings, lectures, and nationwide media appearances, including The Dr. Oz Show, The View, and the Huffington Post. She helps individuals withdraw from substances of abuse, as well as psychiatric medications through the use of specific natural supplements. She has created a unique, high quality line of nutritional supplements for the brain, and is the author of several popular books including Natural Highs, 8 Weeks to Vibrant Health, and The Addicted Brain and How to Break Free. http://www.cassmd.com

If you liked this Amazing Itty Bitty® book you might also enjoy:

- **Your Amazing Itty Bitty® Marijuana Manual** – Kat Bohnsack

- **Your Amazing Itty Bitty® Cancer Book** – Jacqueline Kreple

- **Your Amazing Itty Bitty® Heal Your Body Book** – Patricia Garza Pinto

Or any of the other Amazing Itty Bitty® books available on line.

Made in the USA
Middletown, DE
13 May 2020

94844142R00027